AF255337

5 Polyps Colonoscopy Story

How Ms. Ele Gains Confidence

HILARIOUS COLON PREP

BEFORE

THE EXAMINATION SIDE

Eleanor Lynar

__5 Colonoscopy Story | How Ms. Ele Gains Confidence__ examines through unexpected twist, turns and hilarious humor, how she was determined against all adversity not to fail.

You will learn the importance of a colon screen test that can save your life. It's a nonfiction story in high drama, sequence and conflict…This is her story.

__The 5 Polyps Colonoscopy story | How Ms. Ele Gains Confidence__ is a must read for anyone who may think that this medical examination is not important. It is a primary matter to heed.

Gratification

Eleanor Lynar has been a self-published writer for several years on Amazon online bookstore. She is the author of 7 fiction and 2 nonfiction eBooks. An active reviewer at Fanstory.com and accomplished Poet Laureate.

My satisfying love of words come via Art teacher Ms. Whipple. She played a big role in my childhood maturation. In my later years, Brian Tracy, Jon Franklin, American Writers Association Inc., Amazon Kindle books, as well as so many more.

As for me to write a nonfiction, hilarious book drew from a lifetime of experiences. I owe it all to these people and my God in their training and viewpoints.

Without their friendship and inspiration this book would not have been printed. Anyone reading this book who gains help owe them appreciation.

Eleanor Lynar

Pennsylvania, 2020

Table of Contents

Chapters

I

5 Polyps Colonoscopy Story

November 11, 2019 finds elderly Ms. Ele at home in a struggle to drink down plenty of liquids before her scheduled test.

Two days later, Wednesday afternoon at the College Heights Hospital Center of Pennsylvania is where KH, MD uncovered 5 polyps during the colon examination. This is the story, how Ms. Ele gains confidence.

Just before her procedure, she had a problem drinking 8 fluid ounces every hour for healthy hydration. Then she had to take 3 tiny laxative pills which takes about 3 or 4 hours before a bowel movement.

However, Ms. Ele hears her stomach rumble by 3 hours. She hurries to do number 2 in the toilet. While sitting there she thinks. "Hey, no pain or cramps. This preparation is no sweat."

But little did she know about the explosive force the Golytely intestinal cleaner would exert.

Now it's time for her to drink this mixture every 15 minutes until the bottle is half empty. This would be a problem for Ms. Ele with her Asthma condition.

II: How Ms. Ele Gains Confidence

Still she is determined to cooperate. She gulps, gags, gulps…gags…with a frown face.

The Golytely colon prep worked like a timed bomb as its tic, tic, tics away time. Now before Ms. Ele's next 15-minute drink, she rushes to the bathroom.

Then Boom! The crap hits the toilet bowl sides and water with a Plop..Plop..Plop. Ms. Ele gasped startled!

Afterwards she says, "This stuff works just like a Roto, Rotor repairman, who visits your house who opens a clog drain." The power of Golitely moved the crap, deep inside her intestines, out her anus fast.

Bang zoom, now her bowels were coming so fast she could not reach the toilet seat on time. Well she accidentally soils her bedsheet and Chenille top bedspread. Oh, what a smelly mess. "It's just like oatmeal, mixed with Milk of Magnesia." Ms. Ele screeched!

The worse thing yet, her washing machine had been broken for 1 year. Today, it was not possible for her, to go to the Laundry Mat in her condition. Ms. Ele's mind began to soar like a Bald Eagle.

Quickly she grabs her soiled bed linen to wash by hand. Embarrassed, Ms. Ele forgives her mess.

However, she knew that unforeseen accidents do happen. "It felt awful to have B.M. on her clean bedclothes." She moans.

After she tidy up everything, Ms. Ele gets a light bulb idea. She takes a white plastic garbage liner. Then she cuts it down the middle and cuts off the bottom edge. Next, she opens the bag and she spread it over the bedsheet.

Elated, Ms. Ele discovered how to protect her bedsheet from b.m. stains. Yes, she thinks high 5!

However, all this extra energy has made her very exhausted. So, she decides to take a power nap. Shortly as she dozes, her stomach rumbles and grumbles.

Ut-Oh! While she stands up, some brown stink crap splash on her summer shorts and some stream down her left thigh and lower leg.

"Ah Gut run off." Ms. Ele fumed. Her bowels had turned to pea soup.

Again, she hurries into the bathroom to put her soiled clothes in the sink basin to soak. While there she takes a Lilac Crystal, body bath shower. The bathroom smells great and so does she. Ms. Ele's jangled nerves felt soothe.

II: How Ms. Ele Gains Confidence

This experienced opened her eyes. Where she learned that more faith and endurance was required to stick with the Golitely colon prep.

Now refreshed, Ms. Ele goes back into her bedroom and paused in the doorway. She stares at the Golitely bottle undecided to continue or stop drinking it.

She ponders. Now if this bottle could speak to me, would its mouth reply:

"Hey! Ms. Ele don't blame me for the gut Timed Bomb colon cleaner. Uh-huh, it's very necessary for the test. He-Haw, He-Haw, He-Haw. (laughing) But, remember, you still must drink half the bottle. Golitely tease.

Unphased, Ms. Ele doesn't blink an eyelid. Her resolve is not to fail. She proceeds to gulp and gag down the preparation to the half empty line. Then she put the rest in the refrigerator for later.

She likened her schedule, to a Marathon race in drinking all the fluid down until she reached the finish line. This all helped to demonstrate, how Ms. Ele gain confidence along the way.

5 Polyps Colonoscopy Story

Today is Wednesday afternoon and it's time for the Colonoscopy examination.

While in the hospital bed, Ms. Ele flips through an ELLE magazine. Suddenly her stomach rumbles twice. She must go crap again.

Nurse Karen helps her to the Ladies Room. Once inside, she sits on the toilet to b.m. Unaware, the unfasten hospital gown tail falls into the toilet bowl.

When she stands up, the wet gown drips yellow fluid on the toilet seat, bathroom floor and on her feet. **"Oh, For Crying Out Loud!"** She squeals.

Frantic, she used a soapy towel to wipe clean the toilet seat, floor and used the sink basin to wash her feet. "I don't believe this." She shrieks.

Then she hesitates, before she opens the door with down cast eyes. Now, in a lower self-esteem, she wants to **Vanish**.

Upset, Ms. Ele asked Nurse Karen for a clean gown as she shares her trouble. Tickled, Nurse Karen did all she could do, not to laugh in her face. She imagines the hilarious bathroom scene.

Wounded in spirit, Ms. Ele chose to remain silent while she takes the gown back to her room. She thinks. "For an unexpected blunder, this was it before surgery. **OH, Sweet Apple Cider!** Ms. Ele wail. She was tired of the twists and turns. What else could go haywire now?" she said.

II: How Ms. Ele Gains Confidence

However, the great news was she had a clean intestinal tract. After she saw the yellow return drainage in the toilet bathroom water.

Then she sighs as she rubs lotion on her hands anxious to go, as she waits in bed.

Shortly, Nurse Karen and a staff member roll her into the Surgical Suite. Inside there, she falls into a deep sleep.

She awakes back in her room where the Doctor K. visits to discuss the polyps found and that the results would be faxed to her primary medical doctor's office right away.

Before Ms. Ele leave the hospital, she thanks the doctor and the staff during her short stay.

While outside in the car, her stomach growls like a hungry Black Bear. Her driver and best friend Philomene stop by Chic-fil-A to get her a chicken sandwich before she takes her home. She appreciates Philomene who enjoys helping people by good acts and asking for nothing in return. (neighborly love)

Yes, Ms. Ele would send her a beautiful big nice Gratitude card tomorrow.

Now truth day has arrived, for her doctor's visit. While she waits to see Dr. NG in the examination room, she hears the wall clock tic.. tic.. tic.. as time passes. She sees her life drift away by medical trauma.

Worried, Ms. Ele thinks. What if the 5 polyps test positive for Cancer? Her fears rise. Her older sister had died from stomach cancer… could it be gene related. What type of polyps did she have? Worry questions that her mind ache for answers.

Suddenly, both the palms of her hands became sweaty as her body muscles tensed up. "Oh, hurry doctor, I want to know now!" Nervously, she said.

Next came a tap. tap. tap. on the office door as the doctor enters with my chart in his hands. Ms. Ele braced herself for the truth with a solemn face.

While Dr. N G looks at the report on the office computer, he placed his hand on her left shoulder and said:

"Ms. Ele your 5 polyps, Adenomas were negative for Cancer. But you will have to repeat the Colonoscopy in 3 years, OK?"

II: How Ms. Ele Gains Confidence

"Doc that's if you can catch me." "Hey, that colon prep works like an anus timed bomb!"

Dr. N G replies, "Oh yes, that's what I heard, too smiling. But let's write down that date on both our calendars.

Good idea, she knew the risks for tumors to return. So, she agrees for the follow-up visit.

Relieved, she wipes tears from her eyes; pleased with the results. She thanks him.

In silence, she appreciates that God gave her, a new lease on life. She opens the office door and steps outside into her changed world with insight. Ms. Ele won.

IV: Polyps Colonoscopy Story
Questions About Colonoscopy

How to Head off Colon Polyps

One recent study found that the formation of polyps is unknown, but family genetics play a primary role.

What's amazing is that Medicinenet.com found that polyps are common at **age 60**. Meaning more people are likely to form or get one or more polyps later in life. *Medicinenet.com*. If you would like to Learn more go to their website.

How Fast Do Colon Polyps Grow?

Polyps grow slowly and take years to get big enough to be visible. *HealthTap.com*

Best Food Adjustment for Ms. Ele

She now eats lots of collard green, celery, leaks broccoli, cauliflower, carrots. high fiber cereals, grain breads lentils. Fruits, pineapple, apples, mango, yams.

Her balance exercise with a regular b.m. is very important. Eating less meat and more vegetables and less salt and sugar will help her avoid colon polyps.

II: How Ms. Ele Gains Confidence
Inspirational Quotes

Do you know that the famous Actor and Producer,
Will Smith have this quote to say about his
Colonoscopy?

Will Smith, Producer, Actor

Don't forget to watch his Hilarious Video: IV
Logged My Colonoscopy on You Tube.

Luke Perry, Actor
"So many people could save a life.
If they just go and have a Colonoscopy But you have got to do something."

Brad Field's Businessman
"A rite of passage in America, when you turn 50 and have health insurance is a colonoscopy."

V: Pie Chart Colorectal Polyps

Malignancy Risks:

- Tubular adenoma: 2% @ 1.5 cm – Minhhuyen Nguyen. Polyps of the colon and Rectum, MSD Manual
- Tubulovilbus adenoma: 20% to25 % - (2005). "colorectal Cancer: Epidemiology, Risk Factors and Health Services." Clinics in colon and Rectal Surgery 18.

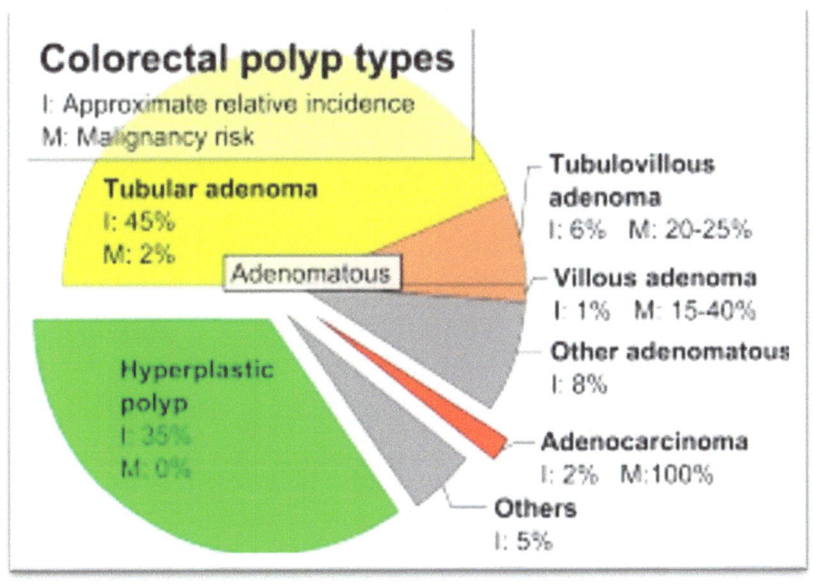

Figure 1-Polyp Chart

The thing is most people know that all foods are healthy to eat. The question remains which foods fight against intestinal polyps? Colorectal polyps act as a parasite in the colon.

So, Ms. Ele faced a major, life changed mindset, when she shopped for food. It was hard. She likes her regular choices. A food switch, at her age, was very uncomfortable. However, she thought deeply about the high-risk factor with the number of polyps that had been removed. Yet, for Ms. Ele, she would not be foolish to hear and not heed her warning signs:

Leafy Harvest Veggies

First, she crossed off her list 3 meat selections. Then they were replaced with collard greens, kale, cabbage, mustard, broccoli, lettuce, spinach, carrots, scallions.

Grain Fiber Choices

Working with her list, she brought oatmeal, grits, brand flakes, almonds, walnuts, wheat bread, beans, brown rice.

Her adjustment would be tough. She ate more meat than a variety of vegetables in her lifetime.

Fruit Medley

Her hands reached for apples, bananas, mangos, oranges, pineapple. When fruit is out of season, she used can fruits instead.

What she also found handy was a food processor to mix, chop, and blend foods. It was easy for her hands with arthritis.

Using Coupons

Although she didn't use coupons, thinking the money saving was not worth it. Oh! How surprised she discover, it wasn't true. When she purchased her vegetables at Produce junction, she got all that she needed, and she saved $8.00 on her order. How neat was that to make ends meet?

This experience made her a believer in using the coupons to afford the adjustment in her diet to prevent polyp formation in the future. She smiles with satisfaction and thanksgiving.

II: How Ms. Ele Gains Confidence
Polyp Prevention Meals

Ms. Ele liked to cook but the problem was her thinking has changed from unhealthy, rich food to a veggie breakfast, dinner and 2 meatless days a week.

The change in diet with a normal regular bowel program, boost her energy. She didn't feel drained out before the end of the day.

She believed that eating junk food without plenty roughage, fiber or grains might have played a large portion in the formation of her colon polyps.

Ms. Ele made an earnest effort to research some satisfying meal selections for her well-balanced gut health in, Food Cures from Reader's Digest.

Her eyes popped wide open. The Western diet she enjoyed – meat, potatoes, enriched white rice, hi-sugar sweets, salt with few veggies for years, failed to promote gut wellness.

What she did learn about hi-fiber foods was that they speed through the intestines. The force doesn't allow polyps to grow or cause trouble in later life.

As she increased the leafy green vegetables like kale, spinach, collard greens, turnip greens that all provide a rich source of vitamins and antioxidants.

What grabbed her was the fresh Pineapple that has the protein enzyme Bromelain to lessen inflammation.

She welcomes this between meal snack. The key is to use only the fresh fruit, not the can or juice type. It keeps you fuller longer. Pineapple helps to decrease the appetite along with helping to calm the stomach. The following picture show what the fresh pineapple looks like.

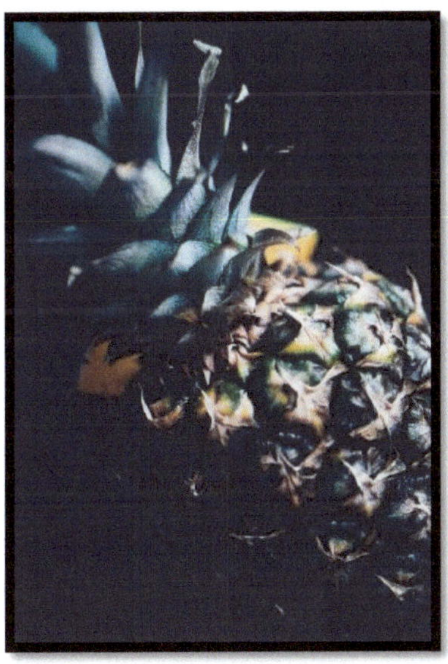

Figure 2-Markus- Pineapple

Now, Ms. Ele did switch the cookies, cakes, candy for wiser healthy food choices for wellness.

II: How Ms. Ele Gains Confidence

What she learned with Garlic it's a powerful antioxidant. Just chopping 1 fresh clove and drinking it with glass of water daily it supports the immune system. The pungent breath aroma is caused by the stomach acid breakdown that cause the bad breath odor. It helps to fight bad bacteria in the gut.

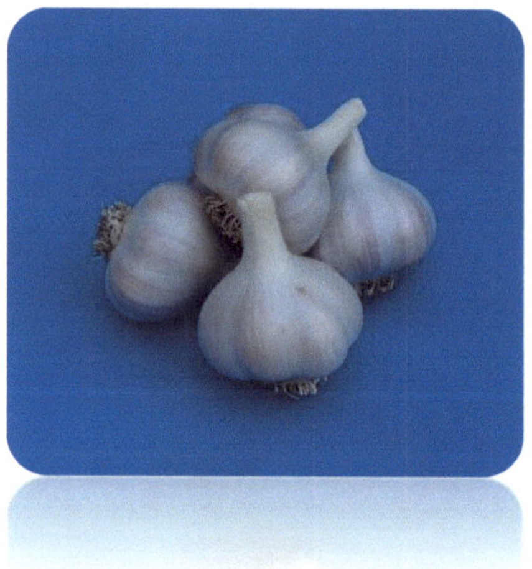

Figure 3-Garlic

She likes to chop a clove of garlic; drink it with water after a meal. It's an immune system booster. For the strong garlic breath. Hot tea with cinnamon, or you can eat a piece of hard mint candy. Check with your doctor first.

Bread and Grain Choices, she had to rearrange her thinking being it's not her favorite items. Later she learned to like oatmeal, grits, corn bread, rye, bran flakes, whole wheat bread, almonds, cashews, pita breads, walnuts, pecans. A variety of hi-fiber, protein healing foods. Whole grain cereals and bread help provide complex carbohydrates can help with poor sleep.

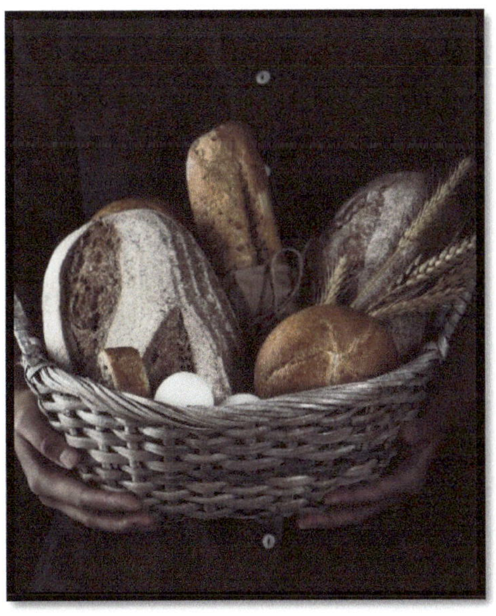

Figure 4- Breads

II: How Ms. Ele Gains Confidence
Bread and Grain Choices

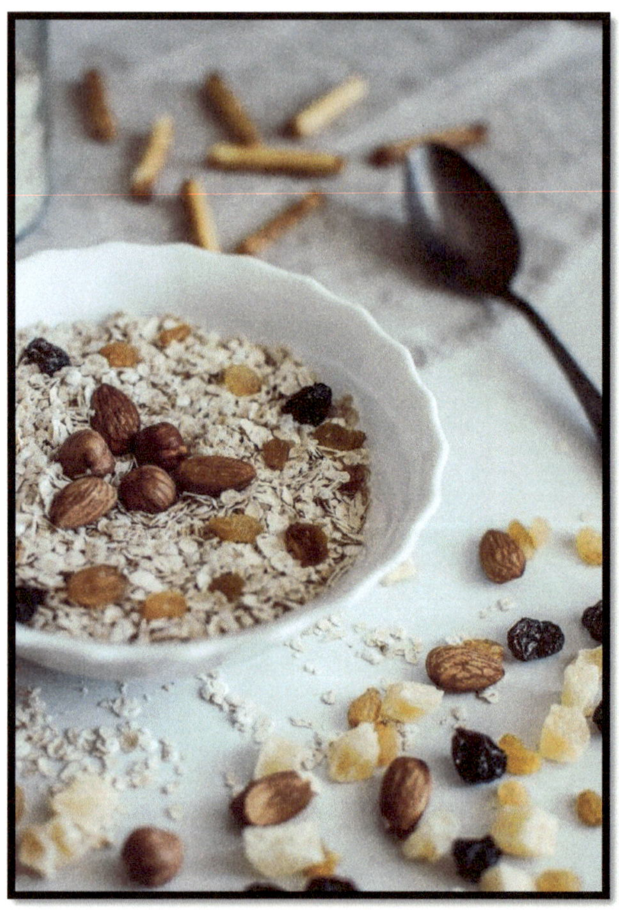

Figure 5-Grains-Nuts

5 Colonoscopy Story

Ms. Ele purchased a food blender for easy quick meal preparation. She had difficulty with the turnkey can opener, chopping veggies or mixing some simple ingredients with her arthritis hands. Her old fashion opener can would open 2 lids then stop working. The electric one wasn't much different too.

However, when the flip top can opener arrived, it was just what she needed. "Bravo!" She said for the inventor.

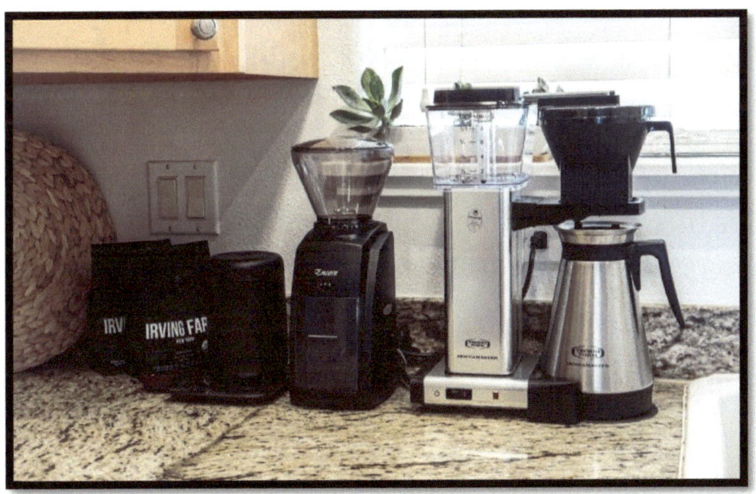

Figure 6-Food Blender

II: How Ms. Ele Gains Confidence
V11: Exercise Reduce Colon Polyps

Researchers found that regular physical exercise was associated with a 16% decrease in the risk of developing colon polyps and with a 30% decrease in the risk of developing large polyps and more likely to become cancerous.
March 9, 2011 www.Medscape.com

Physical exercise early in life prevents colorectal polyps later. It is not uncommon for a specialist Gastroenterologist to find one or two adenomatous during a routine colonoscopy. While these polyps are not cancerous doctors consider them to be cancer forerunners.

Although about half the people aged 60 years or older have them, 6% of the polyps become cancerous. Surgical removal prevents this from happening later. Medical News Today – Newsletter

Ms. Ele Exercises

Now she believed in keeping the body moving with a balance rest periods. She exercises in home and walks outside 10 to 20 minutes two times a day. It helps her digestive tract. She stretches her body limbs to provide more flexibility enduring Arthritis. It gives her an overall sense of well-being.

5 Colonoscopy Story

Next, she takes a deep breath in, holds it for 10 seconds. Then slowly blows the air out through purse lips for 10 seconds.

It helps to air rate her lungs to breathe more easily and to feel more relaxed with Asthma.

Also, she learned that exercise and a good regular bowel schedule will keep the colorectal tract healthy and it will lower polyps' risk. Whereby, exercise helps to rid body waste and it lowers anxiety. After that she feels more energized and ready to do what she wants.

Now what Ms. Ele found was these fascinating quotes that left an echo upon her mind.

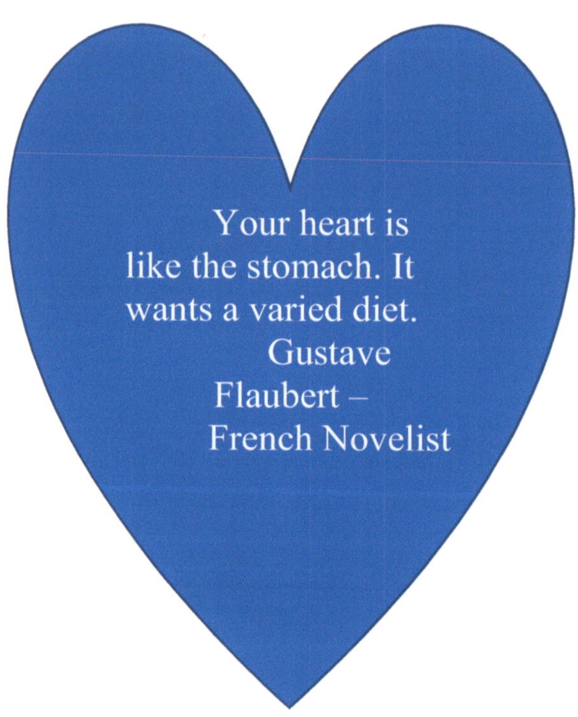
Your heart is
like the stomach. It
wants a varied diet.
Gustave
Flaubert –
French Novelist

"Your diet is like a bank account. Good food choices are a good investment."
Bethenny Frankel – American Businesswoman

The only way to keep your health is to eat what you don't want, drink what you don't like and do what you rather not.
Mark twain – American Author

II: How Ms. Ele Gains Confidence

> "Eating properly is great. You cut the fat down, cut the cholesterol out, but you still get your rest and you now have some form of exercise."
> Mike Ditka – American Coach

Summary

Yes, indeed, Ms. Ele gain confidence when she had the 5 polyps removed by surgery. She changes from an unhealthy Western diet to one with more food cures. There were so many new veggies she didn't have a clue to, which she later enjoyed.

If your doctor recommends a Colonoscopy screen at an earlier age than 50, it would be wise to get it done. Why? Doctors view polyps as a forerunner to colon cancer. By cooperating early cuts, the risk before any intestinal polyp forms.

It is amazing how just a change in the foods that you eat may later save your life. Don't allow the parasite polyp grow on your intestinal track by doing something to prevent them now. Stay healthy.

5 Polyps Colonoscopy Story
Polyp Prevention Veggies

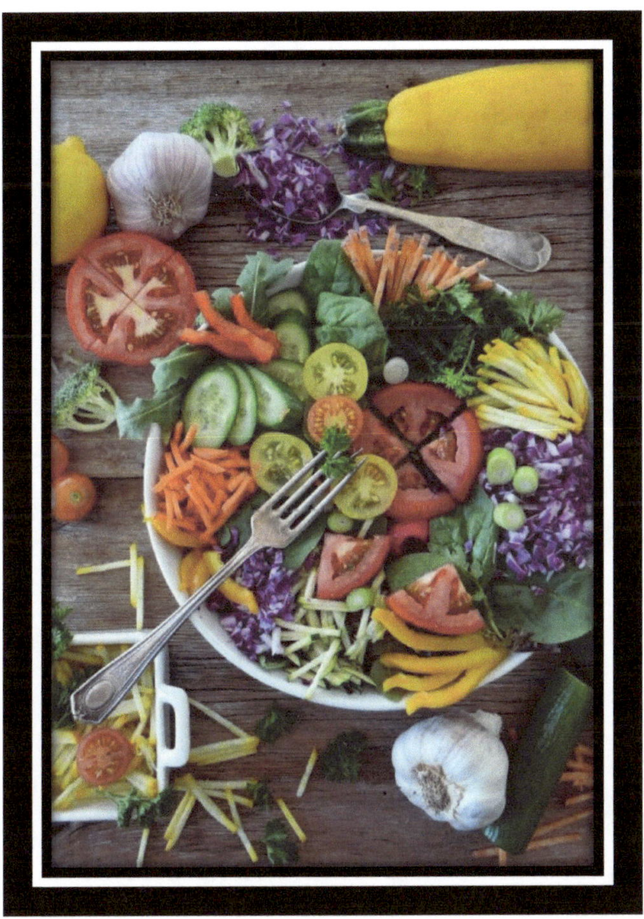

Figure 7-Nadine-Primeau

Vegetable Junction

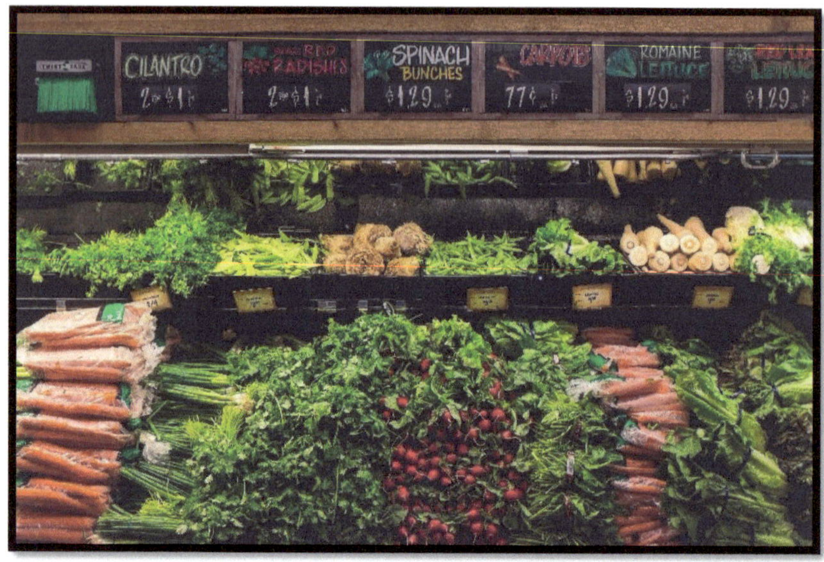

Figure 8-Neonbrand

Notable

It is always better to prevent a health problem early than correct it after it has started. This is like the way it's used in the US.

Benjamin Franklin that said: "An ounce of prevention is worth a pound of cure." He was not talking about food but fire safety. ___Beef Talk